Igor Richter

Rectal cancer

Igor Richter

Rectal cancer

The prognostic significance of change of the epidermal growth factor receptor expression in patients with rectal cancer

LAP LAMBERT Academic Publishing

Impressum / Imprint

Bibliografische Information der Deutschen Nationalbibliothek: Die Deutsche Nationalbibliothek verzeichnet diese Publikation in der Deutschen Nationalbibliografie; detaillierte bibliografische Daten sind im Internet über http://dnb.d-nb.de abrufbar.

Alle in diesem Buch genannten Marken und Produktnamen unterliegen warenzeichen-, marken- oder patentrechtlichem Schutz bzw. sind Warenzeichen oder eingetragene Warenzeichen der jeweiligen Inhaber. Die Wiedergabe von Marken, Produktnamen, Gebrauchsnamen, Handelsnamen, Warenbezeichnungen u.s.w. in diesem Werk berechtigt auch ohne besondere Kennzeichnung nicht zu der Annahme, dass solche Namen im Sinne der Warenzeichen- und Markenschutzgesetzgebung als frei zu betrachten wären und daher von jedermann benutzt werden dürften.

Bibliographic information published by the Deutsche Nationalbibliothek: The Deutsche Nationalbibliothek lists this publication in the Deutsche Nationalbibliografie; detailed bibliographic data are available in the Internet at http://dnb.d-nb.de.

Any brand names and product names mentioned in this book are subject to trademark, brand or patent protection and are trademarks or registered trademarks of their respective holders. The use of brand names, product names, common names, trade names, product descriptions etc. even without a particular marking in this work is in no way to be construed to mean that such names may be regarded as unrestricted in respect of trademark and brand protection legislation and could thus be used by anyone.

Coverbild / Cover image: www.ingimage.com

Verlag / Publisher:
LAP LAMBERT Academic Publishing
ist ein Imprint der / is a trademark of
OmniScriptum GmbH & Co. KG
Heinrich-Böcking-Str. 6-8, 66121 Saarbrücken, Deutschland / Germany
Email: info@lap-publishing.com

Herstellung: siehe letzte Seite /
Printed at: see last page
ISBN: 978-3-659-80705-3

Zugl. / Approved by: Charles university in Prague, 2012

Copyright © 2015 OmniScriptum GmbH & Co. KG
Alle Rechte vorbehalten. / All rights reserved. Saarbrücken 2015

The prognostic significance of change of the epidermal growth factor receptor expression in patients with rectal adenocarcinoma treated with neoadjuvant chemoradiotherapy

Contents

Summary	1
Introduction	4
Epidermal growth factor receptor	4
EGFR and his role in radiotherapy	5
The prognostic significant of EGFR expression in rectal cancer	6
EGFR inhibitors	7
The combination of neoadjuvant chemoradiotherapy and anti-EGFR treatment	8
Material and methods	10
Results	20
Discussion	31
Conclusion	37
References	37

Summary

Aim of the study: The aim of this retrospective study was to determine the prognostic impact of EGFR expression changes during neoadjuvant chemoradiotherapy in patients with locally advanced rectal cancer, by comparision of EGFR expression in pretreatment endoscopical biopsies and resection specimens after neoadjuvant chemoradiotherapy.

Material and methods: Between January 2005 and December 2009 a total of 59 patients were treated with preoperative radiation for rectal adenocarcinoma potentiated with capecitabine in the Department of Oncology, Liberec Hospital. 50 patients, 34 men and 16 women, were evaluated. Nine patients were not evaluated because of incomplete clinical and pathological data. The mean age was 61.4 years (range 40-78 years). Microscopically, tubular adenocarcinoma was identified in all 50 patients. Mucinous component was described in 3 patients. Histologically, the tumour was a well-differentiated adenocarcinoma in 3 patients, moderately differentiated in 38 patients, and poorly differentiated in 9 patients. As far as the anatomical site is concerned, 24 patients had a distal tumour margin localised as far as 5 cm from the internal sphincter, the same number of patients had between 5.1 and 10 cm. The case of the distal edge of the tumour penetrating more than 10 cm was described in 2 patients.

Before the neoadjuvant chemoradiotherapy started, 28 patients were in the second clinical stage and 22 patients in the third clinical stage according to the TNM classification. The source of radiation was a linear accelerator Elekta Precise or Elekta Synergy (Elekta, Sweden). We used ionising photon radiation with the energy of 15 MeV. Patients were irradiated using the 3D conformal radiotherapy technique, or IMRT, using segmented fields. All the patients were administered the total dose of 44 Gy (fractionation of 2 Gy) in 22 fractions to the tumour area, mesorectum and pelvic regional lymph nodes. Capecitabine was concomitantly administered with a dosage of 825 mg/m^2 in two daily oral administrations for the whole duration of radiotherapy including weekends. Surgery was indicated at intervals of 4-8 weeks from the completion of chemoradiotherapy. Imunohistochemical determination of EGFR expression was semi-quantitative and colour intensity of at least 1% of tumour cells was assessed: 0 = none, 1+ = mild, 2+ = moderate, 3+ = severe. The commercial kit (EGFR PharmDx^{TM}, Dako, Denmark) was used. Slides were evaluated by an experienced pathologist who was not familiar with the treatment results of patients. Endobioptic findings before treatment as well as resection specimens after neoadjuvant chemoradiotherapy and surgical treatment were analysed in our patient's group. The statistical evaluation was performed using the Number Cruncher Statistical Systems 9 NCSS (Kaysville, Utah, USA) program. Overall survival (OS) = time from the first histological verification till the death or the date of the last check for survivors. Disease-free survival (DFS) = time from surgery to distant or local recurrence or the last control of a patient without recurrence. The overall survival and disease-free survival was assessed using Kaplan-Meier analysis. The impact of EGFR expression on treatment outcomes (OS, DFS) was assessed by the log -rank test. All the statistical tests were performed at the significance level $\alpha = 0.05$.

Results: All of 50 patients received radiotherapy without interruption up to the total planned dose. No patient died during the treatment. Concomitant chemotherapy was discontinued prematurely in 4 patients because of hematologic and gastrointestinal toxicity. No patient was hospitalized because of acute treatment toxicity. Non-haematological toxicity evaluation did not achieve the grade III or IV. Anaemia grade III was found in one patient. The median time between chemoradiotherapy completion and surgery was 44 days (6.3 weeks). In 30 patients sphincter-saving surgery was performed, 20 patients underwent amputation of the rectum. R0 resection was performed in 47 patients, microscopically positive margin was described by a pathologist in 3 patients. There was no surgically macroscopic residue left in any patient. According to the pathological TNM classification, 14 patients were at the first clinical stage,

24 patients in the second clinical stage and 8 patients in the third clinical stage after the operation. 4 patients achieved complete pathological remission. Complete pathologic response was defined as the absence of tumour tissue in the specimen. No patient had the generalisation of the disease described intraoperatively. Downstaging was described in 30 patients, 26 patients had partial remission. The disease was stable in 15 patients. Progression was reported in 5 patients. At the time of assessment (31 December 2013) was median follow-up 51.3 months. A recurrence was occurred in 25 patients, 25 patients had no signs of recurrence. A local recurrence was found in 8 patients, generalisation of disease was reported in 17 patients. The most common site of metastases were the liver (8 patients) and lungs (7 patients). 1 patient suffered from brain metastases, metastatic involvement of retroperitoneal lymph nodes was found in 1 patient. The median DFS was 64.9 months (95 % CI: 26.1 to 67.8 months). The 3-year DFS was 56 %. A total of 21 patients died, 29 patients remained alive. The median of OS was 76.4 months (95 % CI: 57.3 to 76.9 months). The 3-year OS was 92 %. EGFR expression was examined both by endobiopsy and in resection specimens after neoadjuvant chemoradiotherapy. 46 patients were enrolled into the evaluation of EGFR expression changes. In 4 patients no change expression of EGFR was evaluated because pathologic complete response was achieved after neoadjuvant chemoradiotherapy. Increased EGFR expression was found in 12 patients. In 34 patients no increased expression of EGFR was observed (23 patients without any change of EGFR expression, 11 patients with a decrease of EGFR expression). Statistically significantly shorter OS and DFS was found in patients with increased expression of EGFR compared with patients where no increase expression of EGFR during neoadjuvant chemoradiotherapy was observed. The median OS in patients with increased EGFR expression was 41.1 months (95 % CI 39.1 to 47.0 months). The median OS for patients without the increased expression of EGFR was 76.9 months (95 % CI 76.4 to 76.9 months, log -rank test: $p < 0.0001$). The median DFS in patients with increased EGFR expression was 13.7 months (95 % CI 3.8 to 15.8 months). The median DFS in patients without increased EGFR expression was 67.8 months (95 % CI, 55.7 to 67.8 months, log-rank $p < 0.0001$).

Conclusions: The increase of EGFR expression during neoadjuvant chemoradiotherapy for locally advanced rectal cancer is associated with significant shorter overall survival and disease-free survival.

Introduction

Malignant tumors of the colon and rectum are the most common cancers in developed countries. The incidence of rectal adenocarcinoma represents approximately 30% of this number. For the rectal adenocarcinoma is typical not only the development of the distant metastasis, but the local relapses is presacral area could be described. This fact relates with the anatomical position of rectum in pelvic area. The local relapses are occurred in 5 – 10 % in clinical stage I, in 25 – 30 % in clinical stage II, and in 50 % in clinical stage III [1]. The incidence of local relapses could be reduced by radiotherapy. Metaanalysis of 22 clinical studies demonstrated that neoadjuvant or adjuvant radiotherapy significantly reduced the local relapses incidence compared to surgery alone [2]. A neoadjuvant chemoradiotherapy followed by total mesorectal excision is the current standard of the treatment in patients with locally advanced rectal adenocarcinoma. Neoadjuvant chemoradiation has shown a lower incidence of local recurrence and better toxicity profile compared to adjuvant therapy, but no survival benefit was shown [3, 4]. The combination of radiotherapy with 5-flurouracil (5-FU) or capecitabine has demonstrated a higher number of pathological complete remissions and lower incidence of local relapses compared to the treatment with radiotherapy alone [5 - 7]. The main prognostic factors of rectal adenocarcinoma are clinical stage, radicality of surgery, pretreatment concentration of CEA, tumor grade, angioinvasion, mucinous histology [8]. Epidermal growth factor receptor (EGFR), vascular endotelial growth factor (VEGF), oncoprotein p53, and survivin were studies as the potential new biomarkers for rectal adenocarcinoma [9]. The aim of this retrospective study was to determinate the prognostic impact of epidermal growth factor receptor expression changes during neoadjuvant chemoradiotherapy in patients with locally advanced rectal adenocarcima.

Epidermal growth factor receptor

Epidermal growth factor receptor (EGFR, HER1, erbB-1) is 170 kDa transmembrane glycoprotein [10]. It is composed of 1186 amino acids. The formation of EGFR is encoded by EGFR1 gene, which is localized on the short arm of the chromosome 7 (7p12). EGFR belongs to the erb-B family of the tyrosine kinase receptors. The remaining family members are HER2 (erbB-2), HER3 (erbB-3) a HER4 (erbB-4). EGFR has extracellular ligand-binding domain, a hydrophobic transmembrane domain, and a cytoplasmatic tyrosine kinase domain. [11]. More than 10 ligands are known to bind to the EGFR, including epidermal growth factor (EGF), amphireguline, epireguline, neureguline, transforming growth factor alpha (TGFα), betacellulin, heparin-binding EGF (HB-EGF) [12]. EGFR should by activated by the ionizing radiation too. Ligands binding results in homodimerisation of two EGFR molecules or in heterodimerization of an EGFR molecule with another member of the erbB family. After dimerization and internalisation, autophosphorylation of the intracellular tyrosine kinase domain occur, which activated different intracellular transduction pathways. The results is the cell proliferation, acceleration of cell repopulation, apoptosis inhibition [13]. To the trnaduction pathways belongs Ras/Raf/MAPK, PI3K/AKT, JAK/STAT or PLC/PKC. A major signalling route is the Ras/Raf/MAPK pathway, resulting in increased cell. Another important pathway activates PI3K/AKT, resulting the apoptosis inhibition [13, 14]. EGFR should be directly translocated to the cell nucleus with a direct activation of transcription factors [15 - 18]. EGFR is very important for the reparation of normal epidermal cells. The most important mechanism of the increased activity of EGFR is overexpression in cancer cells. The other mechanisms are increased production of EGFR ligands, activation mutation of EGFR receptor, loss of intracellular regulation mechanisms or EGFR1 gene amplification. The EGFR overexpression is observed in the number of epithelial malignancies. The activation of EGFR on cell surface results with progression of cell cycle, cell proliferation, angiogenesis, apoptosis inhibition. It is also associated with more aggressive properties of cancer cells and resistant to the radiotherapy or chemotherapy [19, 20]. The overexpression of EGFR is responsible for the increased motility of the cancer cells [21].

EGFR and his role in radiotherapy

The reparation, redistribution, repopulation and reoxygenation are the basic mechanisms of interaction between radiation and cells [22]. The EGFR is very important in all this mechanisms. EGFR is important for reparation of the damage cells caused by radiation. EGFR should be directly translocated to the cell nucleus with a direct activation of transcription factors resulting in cells reparation [15 - 17]. Similarly after activation of EGFR caused by radiation results to the activation of Ras/Raf/MAPK pathways with increased of DNA reparation genes (Rad51, ATM, XRCC1) [23, 24]. EGFR has influence for the redistribution of cells after radiation. It was found that EGFR inhibitors cause the redistribution of the cell cycle by G1 phase blockade [25]. Radiobiological studies confirm the critical role of EGFR to cytoprotective and pro-proliferative response of tumour cells after irradiation. The exam mechanism is not fully known. It was found that after application of radiation doses range 1-5 Gy results in immediate activation of EGFR in tumour cells population. After fractionated delivery of 2 Gy was observed overexpression of EGFR which leads to the dose dependent increase of proliferation of the tumour cells [26]. The increase EGFR expression after radiotherapy is related to accelerated repopulation of cancer cells [27, 28]. Increase tumour repopulation during radiotherapy leads to recovery of clonogenic tumour cells, thereby causing counter productivity to radiation therapy alone [29 – 31]. The repopulation of clonogenic tumour cells is therefore undesirable phenomenon in treatment using the radiation. It was studied interaction between EGFR and angiogenesis also. It was observed the inhibition of angiogenesis after incubation of tumour tissue with monoclonal antibody IMC-C225 after EGFR. The decrease expression of vascular endothelial growth factor was observed in this study [32].

The prognostic significant of EGFR expression in rectal cancer

The overexpression of EGFR is observed in 50 – 60 % of rectal carcinoma and is associated with worse prognosis [33 - 35]. Azria evaluated in his study of 77 patients with rectal cancer treated by neoadjuvant radiotherapy the prognostic significance of EGFR expression in pretreatment biopsy. The dose of neoadjuvant radiation was 44 Gy in 22 fractions. In 25 patients with tumour of lower rectum were applied the brachytherapy boost 16 Gy in 2 fractions. The expression of EGFR was observed in 56 % patients. In median of follow-up 36 months was observed significant high number of the local recurrences in patients with overexpression of EGFR above 25 % in multivariate analyse (HR 7.18; $p = 0.037$) [36]. Another study evaluated 92 patients with locally advanced rectal carcinoma treated by neoadjuvant chemoradiotherapy. The EGFR expression was observed in 71 % patients. The patients with overexpression of EGFR had significantly shorter overall survival ($p = 0,013$), significantly shorter disease free survival ($p = 0,002$) and significantly shorter survival without distance metastases ($p = 0,003$) compared with patients without EGFR expression [37]. Giralt in his study presented a total of 87 patients treated for the locally advanced rectal cancer by neoadjuvant treatment. All patients received radiation dose 45 Gy in 25 fractions, 50 patients received chemotherapy. The boost of dose 8 Gy was aplicated in 8 patients. EGFR overexpression was observed in 52 cases (60 % of patients). The patients with overexpression of EGFR had significant less pathological complete response ($p = 0.006$), shorter DFS compared to patients without EGFR overexpression ($p = 0.003$) [38]. EGFR overexpression correlates with the worse prognosis independent of lymph nodes involvement in patients with rectal cancer [38, 39]. Others studies had shown in patients with EGFR overexpression treated by neoadjuvant chemoradiotherapy lower percentage of pCR and shorter DFS [40 – 43]. On the other hand was published retrospective study that have not demonstrated prognostic influence of EGFR overexpression and K-RAS mutation on OS and DFS in 146 patients with rectal cancer treated by neoadjuvant chemoradiotherapy. In this study was EGFR expression evaluated by in situ hybridization [44].

EGFR inhibitors

Based on the above information, the inhibition of EGFR function during cancer treatment is one of the most investigated processes. The two dominant EGFR inhibition strategies under clinical investigation are used [45, 46]. The one group of EGFR inhibitors are small molecules called as tyrosin kinase inhibitors (TKI). TKIs are capable to transit through the cell membrane. Gefitinib (Iressa®) and Erlotinib (Tarceva®) have the greatest importance at now. They are used in treatment in patients with non-small lung cancer as a palliative treatment [47, 48]. This TKIs are not applied in patients with metastatic colorectal cancer. Gefitinib has not demonstrated effect in metastatic colorectal cancer in randomized trial of II phase [49]. Erlotinib also have not demonstrated the efficiancy in monotherapy or in combination with chemotherapy in treatment of metastatic colorectal cancer [50 - 52]. One preclinical study has shown the additive effect of combination of gefitinib, radiotherapy, and chemotherapy [53]. Another clinical study evaluated 41 patients with locally advanced rectal carcinoma. Patients were treated by radiotherapy potentiated by 5-FU and gefitinib. This study demonstrated 30 % of patological complete response (pCR). The problem was higher toxicity of treatment. Gastrointestinal toxicity grade III was observed in 26 % of patients. Gefitinib had to be reduced in 61 % of patients [54]. The another possibility of EGFR inhibition is monoclonal antibodies, that bind to extracelullar domain of EGFR. Cetuximab and panitumumab are the most commonly used in metastatic colorectal cancer. Cetuximab (Erbitux®) is chimeric mouse monoclonal antibodies anti-EGFR that first receiveid US Food and Drug administration aprproval in 2004 for the treatment of irinotecan-refractory colorectal cancer [55]. With the developing of molecular biology was found that important predictive factor for antiEGFR monoclonal antibodies is status of K-RAS gene [56]. K- RAS belongs to the RAS genes family. Another members of RAS genes family are N-RAS and H-RAS genes. The products of RAS genes are regulatory proteins that regulate pathway after EGFR activation. RAS oncogenes are occured in normal unmutated form (wild type) or mutated form with permanent activation regardless of EGFR activation. Mutation of K-RAS gene is observed in 30 – 50 % cases of colorectal cancer. Cetuximab with FOLFIRI regimen showed significant longer PFS and OS in patients with metastatic K-RAS wild type colorectal cancer [57]. Another studies evaluated the effectivness combination of cetuximab and oxaliplatine-based chemotherapy [58 – 60]. Panitumumab (Vectibix®) jis a fully human anti-EGFR antibody. A pilot study showed panitumumab higher effectivness in pretreated patients with metastatic colorectal cancer compared with placebo [61]. Panitumumab was also evaluated in first line traetment in patients with metastatic colorectal cancer with FOLFOX regimen. The best results were observed in the group of patients with wild type of RAS genes. In this group patients was the OS prolonged by 6 months compared with patients with chemotherapy alone [62]. Mutation of N-RAS gene is obsrved in v 5 % of cases. The status of RAS gene is predictive factor for using of antiEGFR antibodies in metastatic colorectal cancer treatment at now. The prognostic significance of K-RAS gene is not clear today [63, 64].

The combination of neoadjuvant chemoradiotherapy and anti-EGFR treatment

Monoclonal anti-EGFR antibodies has shown efficiency in the treatment of metastatic colorectal cancer. Neoadjuvant treatment of rectal cancer has been the topic of several clinical studies I/II phases evaluating the benefits of monoclonal antibodies against EGFR combined with chemotherapy. The chemotherapy regimens included of 5-FU, capecitabine, oxaliplatine or irinotecan. The dose of radiation were in range 45 – 50.4 Gy. The primary point was number of pathological completed response as the predictor of longer DFS and OS [65 – 68]. Most dates are for cetuximab than panitumumab. Eleven clinical studies showed average numebr of pCR only 10.7 % (range 0 – 25 %) of cases (table 1) [69 – 79]. On other side, the percentage of pCR in separate chemoradiotherapy was 13.5 % in 3157 patients in metaanalysis of clinical studies II/III phase [80]. The occurrence of toxicity grade III/IV was described in 30 % in combination of neoadjuvant chemotherapy and cetuximab. The most common was diarrhea, less frequnetly been observed leucopenia, anemia, elevation of liver transaminases. The acneiformic rash was observed in 87 % of cases, but predominantly in grade I/II. Hypersenzitiation reaction after infusionla aplication of cetuximab were observed in 5 – 10 % of cases.

Table 1. Study evaluated pathological complete response (%) in patients treated by chemoradiotherapy and cetuximab.

Studie	N	Cetuximab	Capecitabin	5-FU	Oxaliplatine	Irinotecan	pCR (%)
Chung	20	+	-	+	-	-	12

Author	N						pCR %
[69]							
Machiels [70]	40	+	+	-	-	-	5
Rodel [71]	48	+	+	-	+	-	8
Hoffheinz [72]	20	+	+	-	-	+	25
Horisberger [73]	50	+	+	-	-	+	8
Bertolini [74]	40	+	-	+	-	-	7.5
Hong [75]	10	+	+	-	-	+	20
Cabebe [76]	23	+	+	-	First 10 patients	-	17
Eisterer [77]	28	+	+	-	-	-	0
Velenik [78]	37	+	+	-	-	-	8,1
Kim [79]	40	+	+	-	-	+	23

Panitumumab was evaluated in neoadjuvant treatment of rectal cancer with chemotherapy and radiotherapy in clinical study II phase. A total of 60 patients were treated. The number of pCR was 21 % of cases [81]. On the basis of results of studies evaluating the role of antiEGFR antibodies in neoadjuvant treatment of rectal cancer, this approach is not as standard. It seems that the results of combination cetuximab and chemotherapy in metastatic colorectal cancer or combination of cetuximab and radiotherapy in locally advanced squamous cell carcinoma of the head and neck we cannot to interpolate to the neoadjuvant treatment of locally advaced rectal cancer [55 – 62, 82]. Some studies evaluated the prognostic significant of K-RAS mutation status in neoadjuvant treatment of rectal cancer. Already mentioned study evaluated the influence of panitumumab in neoadjuvant tratment of rectal cancer has not shown the prognostic significant of K-RAS gene mutation state and response rate [81]. The EXPERT study evaluated a total of 161 patients with locally advanced rectal cancer. The treatment was consist of combination of neoadjuvant chemoradiotherapy (potenciated by capecitabine) and CAPOX regimen before and after chemoradiotherapy for both study arm. Cetuximab have been aplicated in one arm in all phases of treatment. The patients with wild type K-RAS treated with cetuximab has shown longer OS (HR 0.27; p=0.034) compared with patients without cetuximab [83]. The following study demostrated the higher percentage of pCR (37 % versus 11 %) in patients in wild type K-RAS compared to mutation K-RAS status. A total of 39 patients with locally rectal cancer were treated with neoadjuvant chemoradiotherapy and cetuximab. Muation K-RAS status were observed in 6 patients, 30 patients had wild-type K-RAS gene [84]. On the other hand some studies has not shown prognostic influence of mutation status of K-RAS gene [75, 85]. An interesting fact is the lower incidence mutation K-RAS status in rectal carcinoma (12 – 30 %) compared to colon carcinoma [86, 87]. The results of studies evaluated the influence of anti-EGFR antibodies with the combination of neoadjuvant chemoradiotherapy for recta cancer are not ideal [69 – 79]. The more options of how to better individualise the treatment of patients with EGFR inhibitors are being looked for. One of them is the research about the dynamics of EGFR expression during the neoadjuvant chemoradiotherapy. This topics was the main aim our study.

Material and methods

Between January 2005 and December 2009 a total of 59 patients were treated with neoadjuvant chemoradiotherapy for rectal adenocarcinoma in our Department of Oncology. Fifty patients (34 men and 16 women) were evaluated. Nine patients were not evaluated because of incomplete clinical and pathological data. The median age was 61.4 years (range 40 – 78 years). Twenty-eight patients had clinical stage II and 22 patients had clinical stage III tumour. The anatomical localization was as follows: 24 patients lower rectum (< 5 cm from the anal verge), 24 patients middle rectum (> 5 – 10 cm), and 2 patients upper rectum (above 10 cm from the anal verge). All patients had a histologically verified adenocarcinoma in a pretreatment biopsy: 3 patients grade I, 38 patients grade II, and 9 patients grade III. Mucinous component was described in three patients. The median of pretreatment concentration of hemoglobine was 142.5 (79 – 166) g/L, leukocytes 8.1 (3.5 – 13.5) * 10^9/L, and thrombocytes 260 (146 – 440) * 10^9/L. Pretreatment concentration of CEA was evaluated in 29 patients. Median CEA level was 3.2 (0.5 – 377) µg/L. Eleven patients had the elevation of CEA.

Treatment

Neoadjuvant treatment consisted of external beam radiation and chemotherapy. The source of radiation was a linear accelerator Elekta Precise or Elekta Synergy (Elekta, Sweden). The photon energy was 15 MeV. Patients were treated in supine position with fully bladder (Fig 1). The localization held on RTG simulator with AP projection. Then patients absolved the planning CT with reconstruction of slices of thickness of 5 mm. The contouring of targeted volumes and organs at risk was performed by planning system PrecisPlan 2.15 (figure 2). Patients were irradiated by 3D conformal radiotherapy technique, or IMRT using segmented fields (figure 3). A total dose of 44 Gy in 22 fractions (single dose 2 Gy) was administered. The target volume consist of rectum with tumour, mesorectum and pelvic regional lymph nodes. All patients were treated by using one targeted volume. The organ at risk were bladder and bowel sac. The verification was once of week with the help cone-beam CT or portal image. Capecitabine was concomitantly administered with a dosage of 825 mg/m2 in two daily oral administrations for whole duration of radiotherapy, including weekends. Surgery was performed 4 – 8 weeks after end of chemoradiotherapy.

Figure 1. Supine position in irradiated patient in our departmend of Oncology

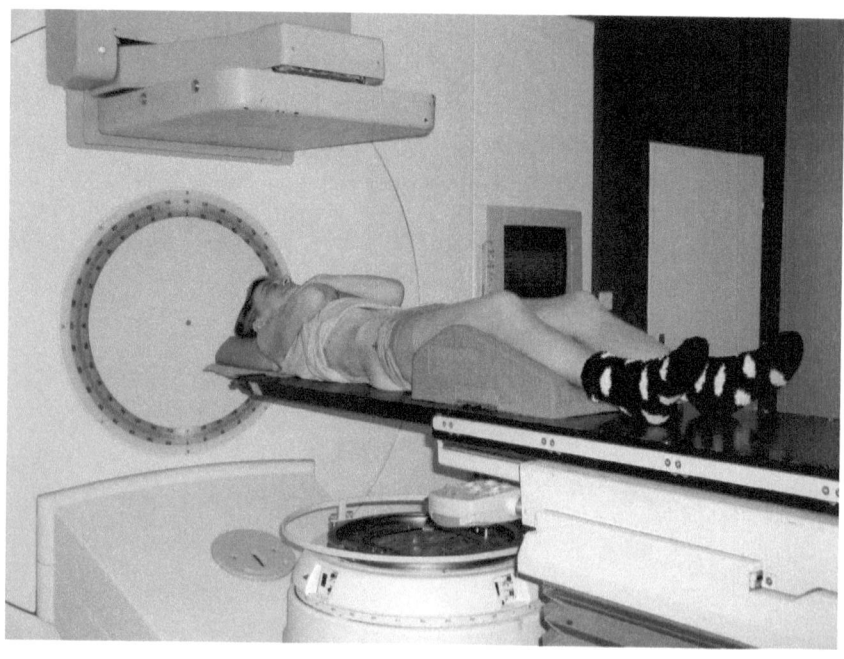

Figure 2. Targeted volumes in radiotherapy of rectal cancer

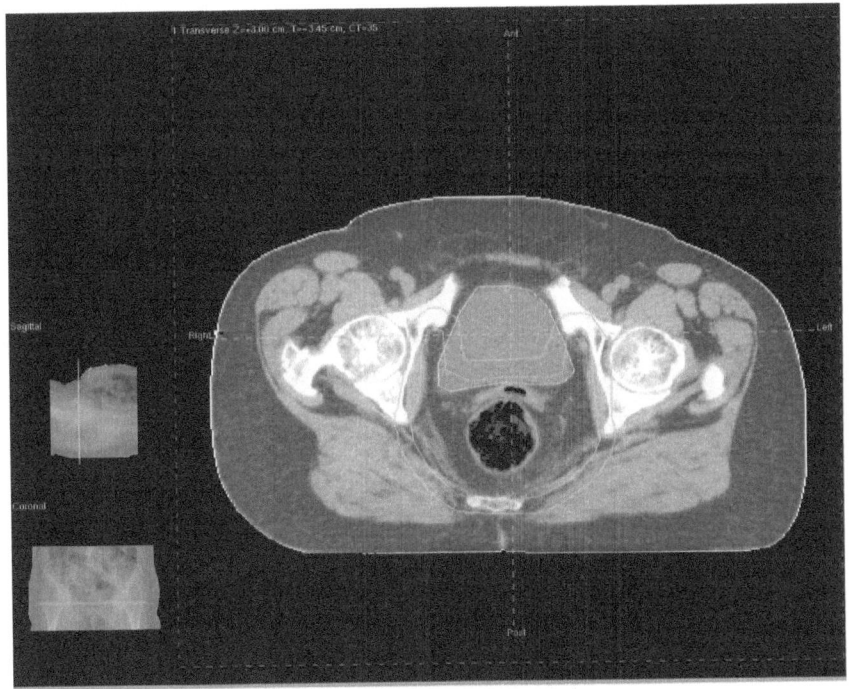

Figure 3. Isodose plane of the radiotherapy of rectal cancer

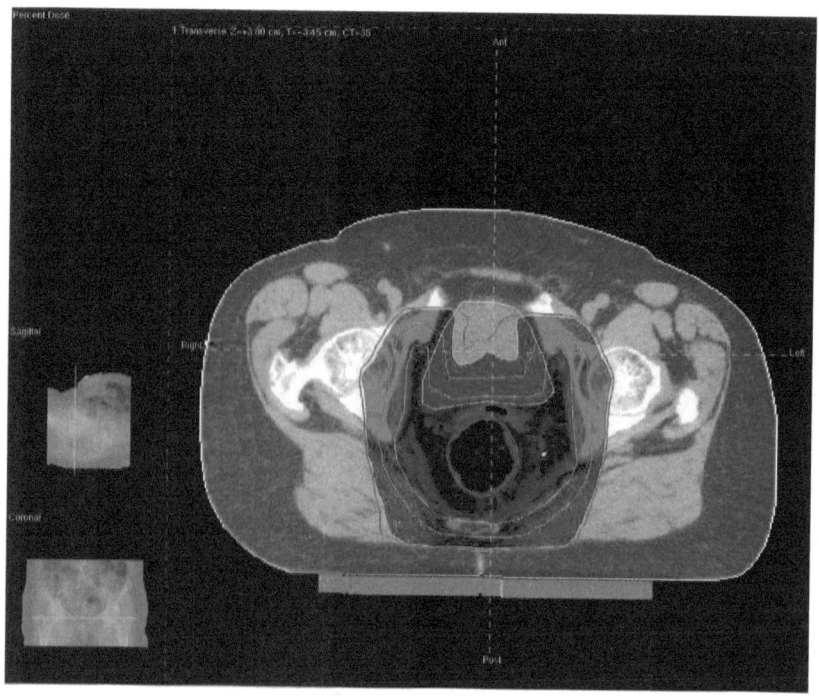

Immunohistochemical determination of EGFR

Routinely fixed, paraffin-embedded blocks of pretreatment biopsies and resected specimens were cut in 3 μm sections. Slides were deparafinized with xylene and rehydrated, and subsequently treated with proteinase K for antigen retrieval. Endogenous peroxidase activity was blocked with Peroxidase Block solution with 3% hydrogen peroxide. Sections were incubated in complete medium for 30 min at room temperature with EGFR pharmDx monoclonal mouse anti-human IgG1 antibody (EGFR pharmDxTM, DakoCytomation, Denmark). A labelled polymer-HRP was then applied and incubated for 30 min. DAB+ substrate-chromogen solution was used for visualization after 10 min incubation, after which slides were counterstained with hematoxylin. As a control for EGFR expression, EGFR pharmDx control slides containing section of two pelleted, formalin fixed, paraffin-embedded human cell lines were used: one representing a moderate level of EGFR protein expression and the other no EGFR expression. Specimens were examined under light microscope. All slides were assessed for EGFR expression by a trained pathologist who was blinded for tumour response data. The evaluation was semi-quantitative as the colour intensity of at least 1% of tumour cells was assessed as follow: 0 = none, 1+ = mild, 2+ = moderate, 3+ = strong (figures 4 – 7).

Figure 4. EGFR score 0. Magnificance 200x.

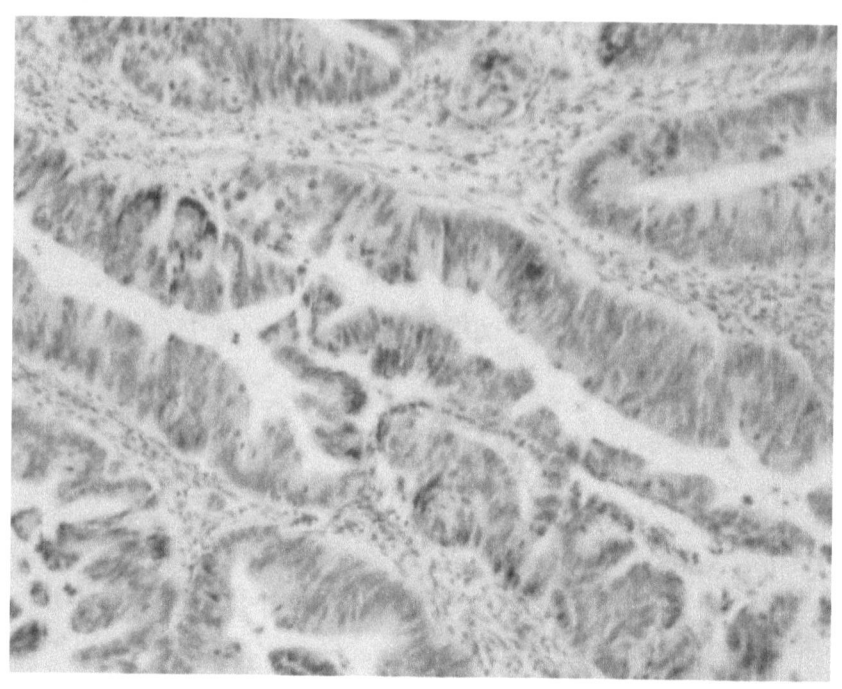

Figure 5. EGFR score 1+. Magnificance 200x.

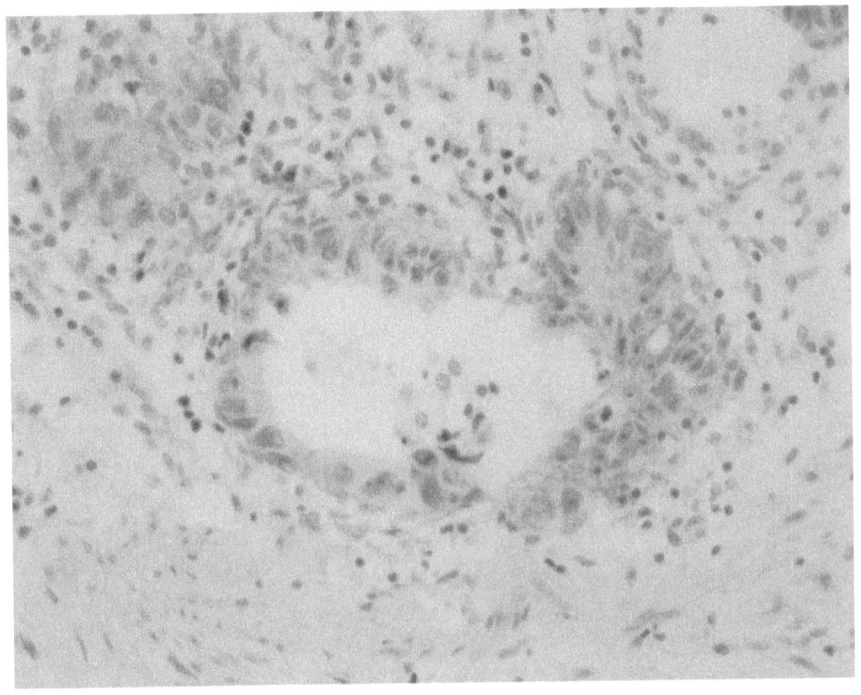

Figure 6. EGFR score 2+. Magnificance 200x.

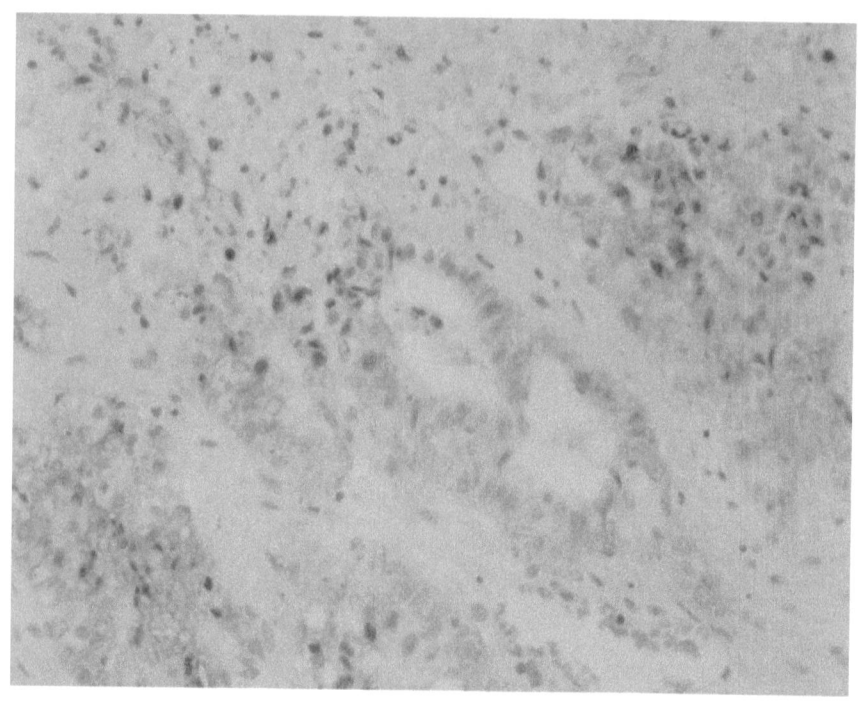

Figure 7. EGFR score 3+. Magnificance 200x.

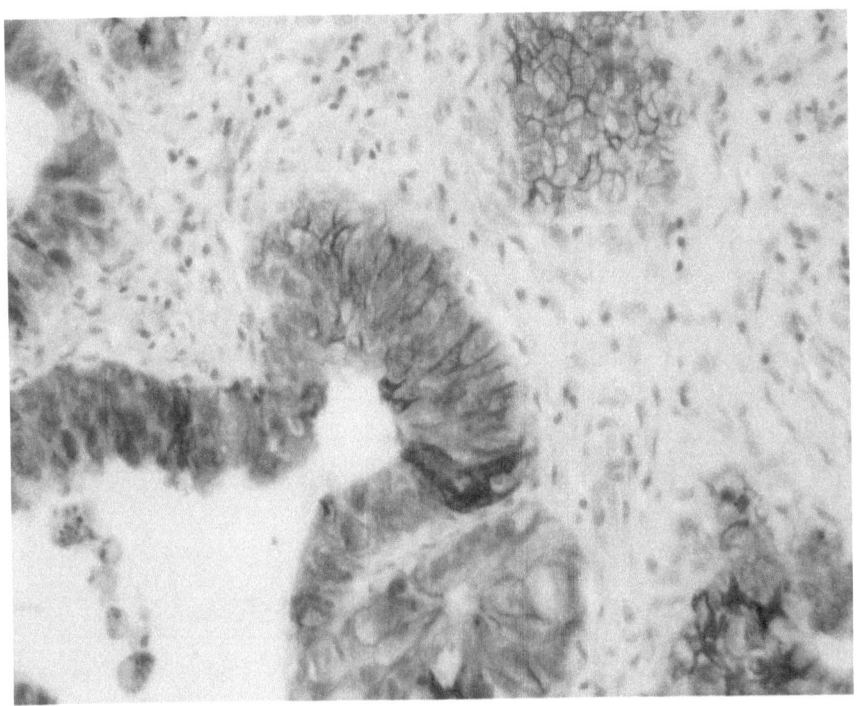

Statistical analysis methods

Disease-free survival (DFS) and overall survival (OS) were counted from the date of the star therapy and analysed using the Kaplan-Meier method. Relationship between the level of EGFR expression and clinical/histopathologic characteristic were analysed using the chi^2 test. Fisher exact test was used on a four-field table when the number of cases was fewer than 10. The prognostic significance of EGFR expression in biopsies and resected specimens and prognostic significance of increase EGFR expression during neoadjuvant chemoradiotherapy on treatment outcomes was assessed by the log-rank test. Multivariate analysis was performed using the Cox regression. We considered $p < 0.05$ to be statistical significant. All statistical analyses were performed using the NCSS 9 statistical software program (NCSS, USA).

Results

All of 50 patients received radiotherapy without interruption up to the total planned dose. No patient died during the treatment. Concomitant chemotherapy was discontinued prematurely in 4 patients because of hematologic and gastrointestinal toxicity. No patient was hospitalized because of acute treatment toxicity. Non-hematological toxicity evaluation did not achieve the grade III or IV. The most common type of toxicity were gastrointestinal complains observed in 44 patients, of them 16 have had nausea and vomiting grade I or II. Hematological toxicity in general was expressed in 25 patients. Anemia grade I was found in 9 patients, grade II in 10 patients, grade III in one patient. Grade I leukopenia was found in 11 cases, grade II in 2 patients. One patient has had a grade II thrombocytopenia. The median of hemoglobin nadir was 115.5 g/L, leukocytes nadir $4.55*10^9$/L, platelet nadir $182.5*10^9$/l. We described the malignant melanoma in one patient with early dissemination. Melanoma was localized out of the irradiated area.

Surgery was indicated in all the patients following 4-8 weeks from neoadjuvant chemoradiotherapy completion. The median time between chemoradiotherapy completion and surgery was 44 days (6.3 weeks). In 30 patients sphincter-saving surgery was performed, 20 patients underwent amputation of the rectum. No patient was assessed by the surgeon and found inoperable. R0 resection was performed in 47 patients, microscopically positive margin was described by a pathologist in 3 patients. No patient was left surgically macroscopic residue. According to the pathological TNM classification, 14 patients were postoperatively at the first clinical stage, 24 patients in the second clinical stage and 8 patients in the third clinical stage. In 4 patients achieved pCR. Downstaging was described in 30 patients. Progression was reported in 5 patients. At the date of analysis was median follow-up 51.3 months.

Overall survival

To the date of analysis died 21 patients, 29 were alive. The median of OS was 76.4 months (95% CI: 57.3 – 76.9). The 3-year OS evaluated in all patients was 92 % (fig. 8).

Figure 8. Overall survival (in months) in patients treated by chemoradiotherapy for rectal cancer

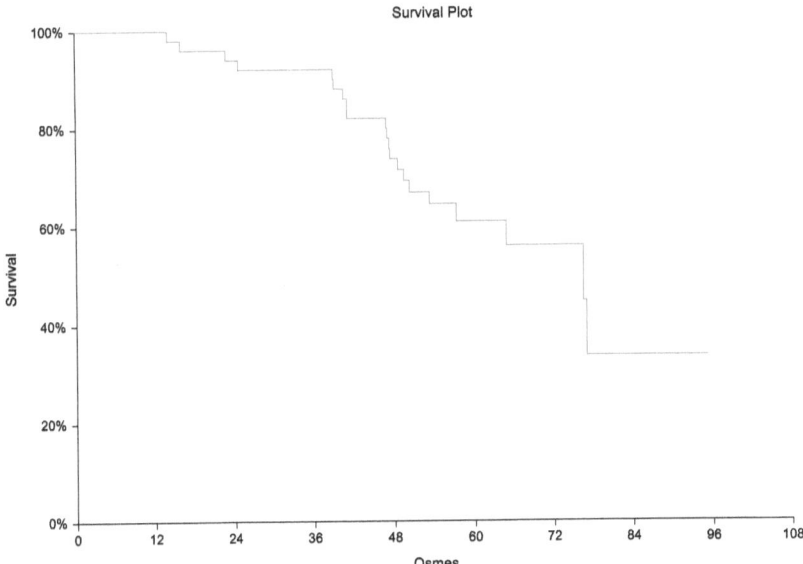

Disease free survival

At the time of assessment a recurrence occurred in 25 patients, 25 patients had no signs of recurrence. A local recurrence was found in 8 patients, generalization of disease was reported in 17 patients. The most common site of metastases was the liver (8 patients) and lungs (7 patients). 1 patient suffered from brain metastases, metastatic involvement of retroperitoneal lymph nodes was found in 1 patient. The median of DFS was 64.9 months (95% CI 26.4 – 67.8). The 3-year DFS evaluated in all patients was 56 % (fig. 9).

Figure 9. Disease free survival (in months) in patients treated by chemoradiotherapy for rectal cancer

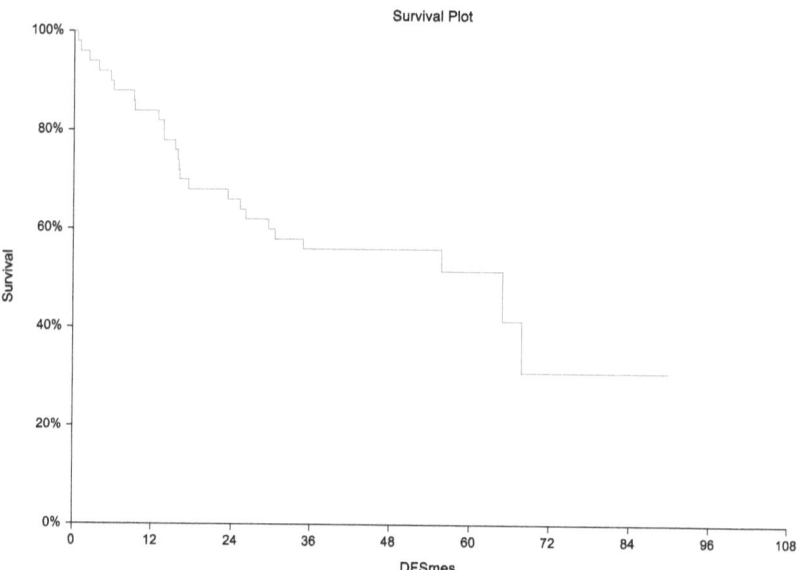

EGFR expression

EGFR expression was examined both by endobiopsy and in surgical resection after neoadjuvant chemoradiotherapy. Endobiopsy EGFR was examined in all 50 patients. EGFR 1 + was observed in 18 patients, EGFR 2 + in 5 patients and EGFR 3 + in 5 patients. Overall, EGFR expression was detected in 28 patients. 22 patients were not detected EGFR expression in endobiopsy. EGFR expression was examined and evaluated in 46 patients in the resection. In 4 patients, EGFR expression not was examined in resection because pCR after neoadjuvant chemoradiotherapy has been achieved. EGFR 1 + was found in 8 patients, EGFR 2 + in 11 patients and EGFR 3 + in 4 patients. Overall, EGFR expression was detected in 23 patients. In 23 patients, no expression of EGFR was detected in the resection. 46 patients were enrolled into the evaluation of EGFR expression changes. In 4 patients no change expression of EGFR evaluated because it was achieved pCR after neoadjuvant chemoradiotherapy. Increased EGFR expression was found in 12 patients. In 34 patients no increased expression of EGFR was observed (23 patients without any change of EGFR expression, 11 patients with a decrease of EGFR expression, table 2).

Table 2. EGFR expression changes in patients in our study

	Počet pacientů
EGFR – incresed	12
EGFR – without changes	23
EGFR – decrease	11

The intensity of EGFR expression in biopsies before treatment had no significant impact on OS and DFS. The median of OS in patients with EGFR expression in biopsies was 76.9 months (95% CI 49.4 – 76.9). Median of OS in patients without EGFR expression in biopsies was 76.4 months (95% CI 53.3 – 76.4). Log-rank: p = 0.9676 (fig. 10). The median of DFS in patients with EGFR expression in biopsies was 55.7 months (95% CI 17.4 – 55.7). Median of DFS in patients without EGFR expression in biopsies was 64.9 months (95% CI 23.3 – 67.8). Log-rank: p = 0.9837 (fig. 11).

Figure 10. Overall survival (in months) in patients with EGFR expression (full line) and in patients without EGFR expression (dotted line) in pretreatment specimen

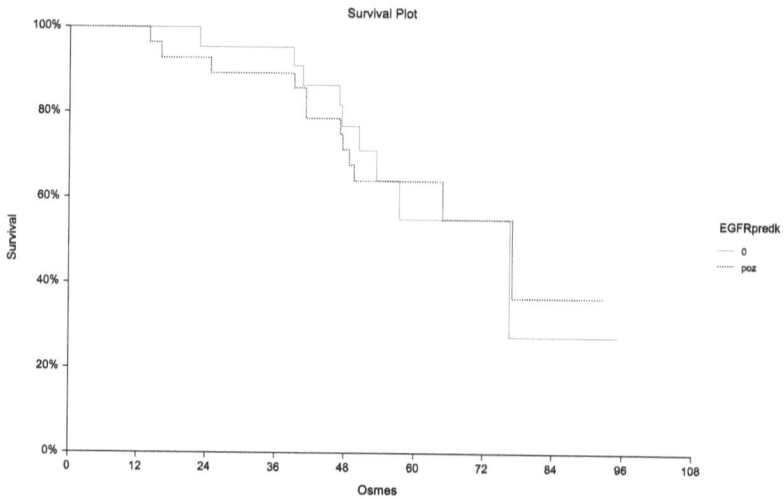

Figure 11. Disease free survival (in months) in patients with EGFR expression (full line) and in patients without EGFR expression (dotted line) in pretreatment specimen

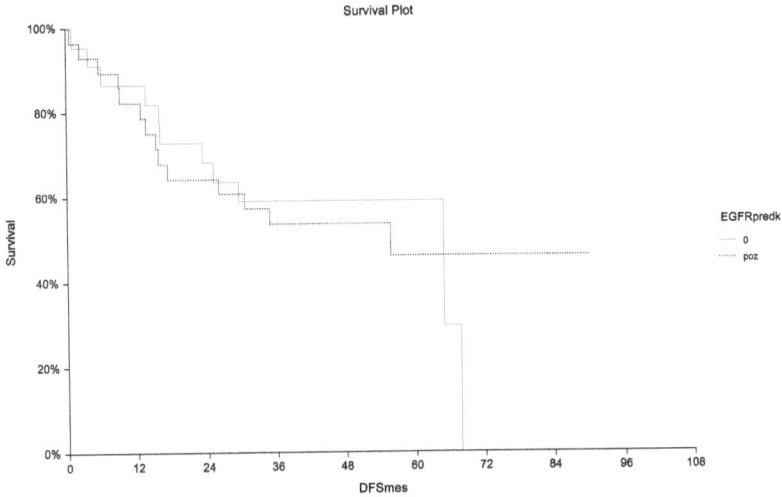

The intensity of EGFR expression in resected specimens after treatment had significant impact on OS and DFS. The median of OS in patients with EGFR expression in resected specimens was 49.4 months (95% CI 41.1 – 64.8). Median of OS in patients without EGFR expression in resected specimens was 76.9 months (95% CI 76.4 – 76.9). Log-rank: p = 0.001

(fig. 12). The median of DFS in patients with EGFR expression in resected specimens was 23.3 months (95% CI 13.7 – 34.8). Median of DFS in patients without EGFR expression in resected specimens was 67.8 months (95% CI 55.7 – 67.8). Log-rank: p = 0.0032 (fig. 13).

Figure 12. Overall survival (in months) in patients with EGFR expression (blue line) and in patients without EGFR expression (red line) in resected specimen

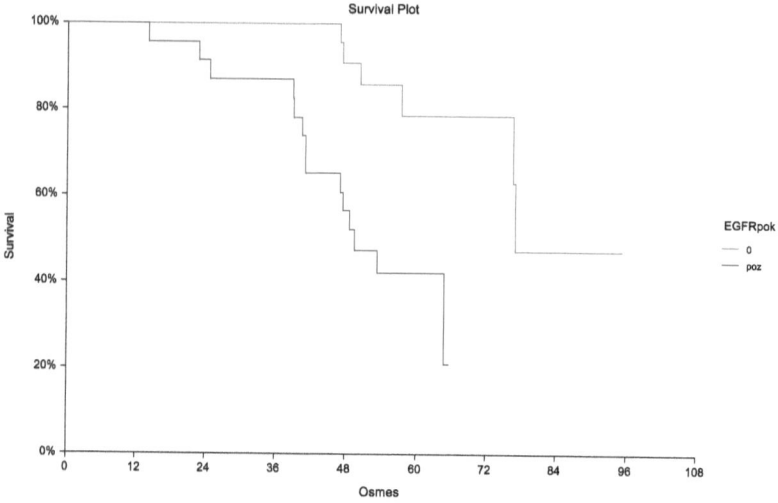

Figure 13. Disease free survival (in months) in patients with EGFR expression (blue line) and in patients without EGFR expression (red line) in resected specimen

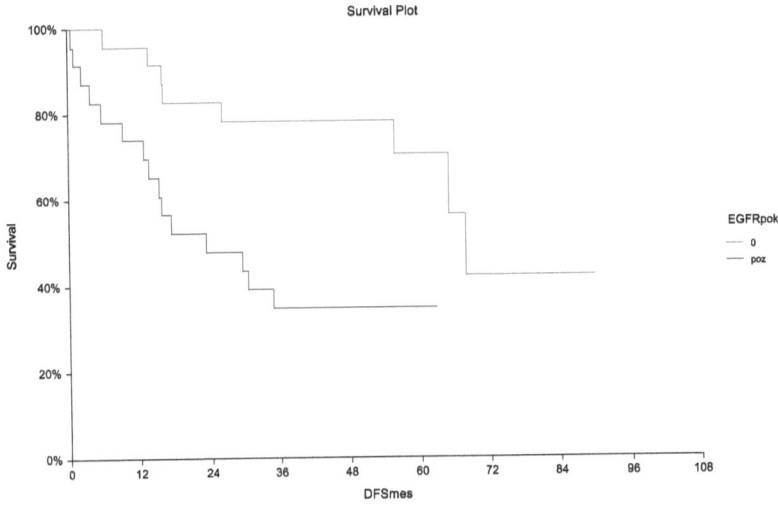

The increase of EGFR expression during neoadjuvant treatment had significant impact on OS and DFS. The median of OS in patients with increase of EGFR expression was 41.1 months (95% CI 39.1 – 47.0). Median of OS in patients without increase of EGFR expression was

76.9 months (95% CI 76.4 – 76.9). Log-rank: p < 0.001 (fig. 14). The median of DFS in patients with increase of EGFR expression was 13.7 months (95% CI 3.8 – 15.8). Median of DFS in patients without increase of EGFR expression was 67.2 months (95% CI 55.7 – 67.8). Log-rank: p < 0.001 (fig.15).

Figure 14. Overall survival (in months) in patients with increased EGFR expression (blue line) and patients without increased EGFR expression (red line) after chemoradiotherapy

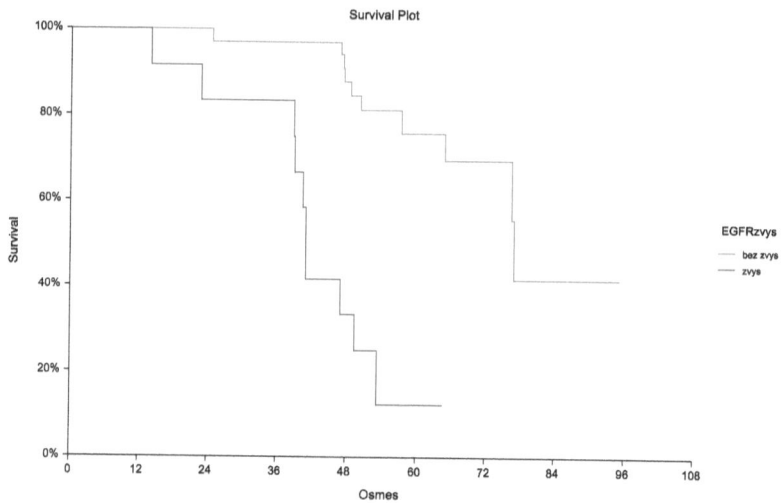

Figure 15. Disease free survival (in months) in patients with increased EGFR expression (blue line) and patients without increased EGFR expression (red line) after chemoradiotherapy

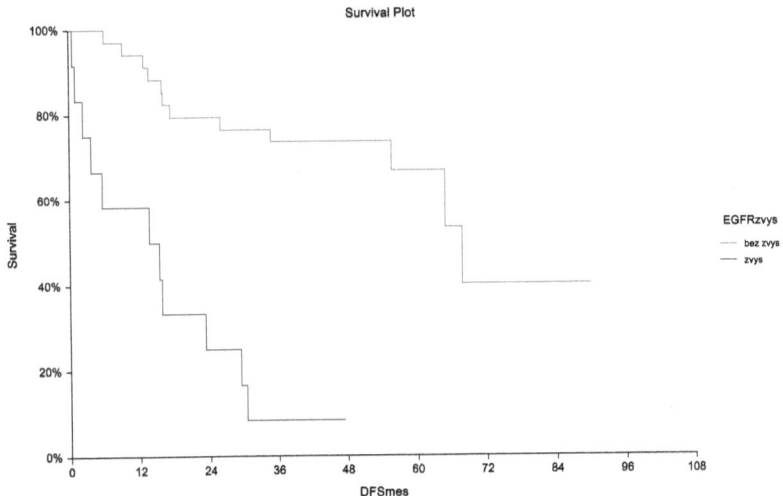

Multivariate analysis

Multivariate analysis was performed using the Cox regression. The significant positive influence to OS were following factors: downstaging, female gender, sphincter saving surgery. The significant negative influence to OS were following factors: EGFR expression in pretreatment biopsy and resected specimens (tab. 3).

Table 3. Multivariate analysis factors on overall survival (thick fon – statistically significance).

Prognostic factor	p-value	Risk ratio	95% CI
Downstaging	**0,0422**	30,68	0,94 – 1000,71
Tumor grade	0,1158	14,37	0,75 – 275,52
Sex	**0,0005**	100,01	5,18 – 1929,43
Clinical stage	0,0579	0,091	0,006 – 1,34
Pathological stage	0,0902	7,907	0,24 – 259.91
Localization of tumour	0,2483	7,046	0,56 – 87,48
Start value of hemoglobine	0,1123	0,954	0,89 – 1,0125
EGFR expression in biopsy	**0,0156**	0,082	0,008 – 0,78
EGFR expression in resected specimen	**0,0001**	1336,817	35,05 – 10000,0
Sphincter saving surgery	**0,0279**	0,052	0,0031 – 0,8608

Discussion

The results of the present study demonstrated significantly inferior DFS and OS in patients with tumors that had increased EGFR expression after neoadjuvant chemoradiotherapy. The increase EGFR expression after radiotherapy is related to accelerated repopulation of cancer cells [27, 28]. Increase tumour repopulation during radiotherapy leads to recovery of clonogenic tumour cells, thereby causing counter productivity to radiation therapy alone [29 – 31]. The repopulation of clonogenic tumour cells is therefore undesirable phenomenon in treatment using the radiation. We demonstrated increase expression of EGFR in 12 patients, i.e. 26.1 % of all evaluated patients. In 2012 was published a retrospective study in 53 patients with locally advanced rectal cancer treated by neoadjuvant chemoradiotherapy. The aim of study was similar with the presented study. During chemoradiotherapy 14 patients (26 %) had an increase EGFR expression. Patients with increased EGFR expression during treatment had significantly shorter DFS (HR 3.02, 95% CI 1.15 – 7.98, p = 0.003) and OS (HR 2.86, 95% CI 1.10 – 7.40, p = 0.005) than patients with either no change or decreased EGFR expression. In this study patients were treated with radiotherapy (total dose 50.4 Gy) and chemotherapy (continual administration of 5-FU) [88]. Both studies demonstrated the prognostic influence of change of EGFR expression on DFS and OS in two different groups of patients treated in two different cancer centres. EGFR was evaluated in different pathology laboratories. In the group of 53 patients, radiotherapy was potentiated by continuous 5-FU, and in our group by capecitabine. In both studies the prognostic significant of EGFR dynamics was confirmed, therefore they cannot be considered to be pure coincidence but a proven link. In 2014 we published the summary analysis of both above studies with actually follow-up. A total of 103 patients were evaluated. In patients without increasing of EGFR expression was significantly longer DFS (HR 3.51, 95% CI 1.62 – 7.61, p < 0.0001) and OS (HR 3.40, 95% CI 1.64 – 7.04, p < 0.0001, OBR) compared with patients with increased of EGFR. The patients with increase of expression of EGFR had significantly porter 5-years DFS (20.9% versus 63.3%, p < 0.0001) and OS (23.3% versus 68.8%, p < 0.0001) compared with patients with either no change or decreased EGFR expression (fig 16 and 17) [89].

Figure 16. Overall survival (in months) in patients with increased EGFR expression (dotted line) and patients without increased EGFR expression (full line) after chemoradiotherapy

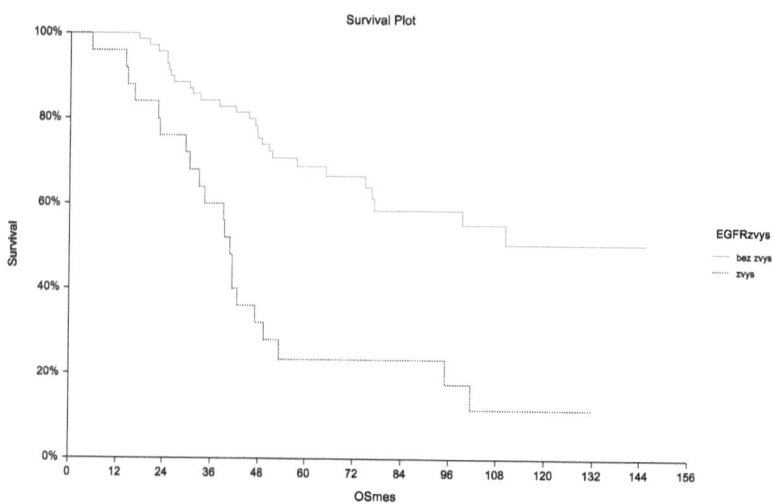

Figure 17. Disease free survival (in months) in patients with increased EGFR expression (dotted line) and patients without increased EGFR expression (full line) after chemoradiotherapy

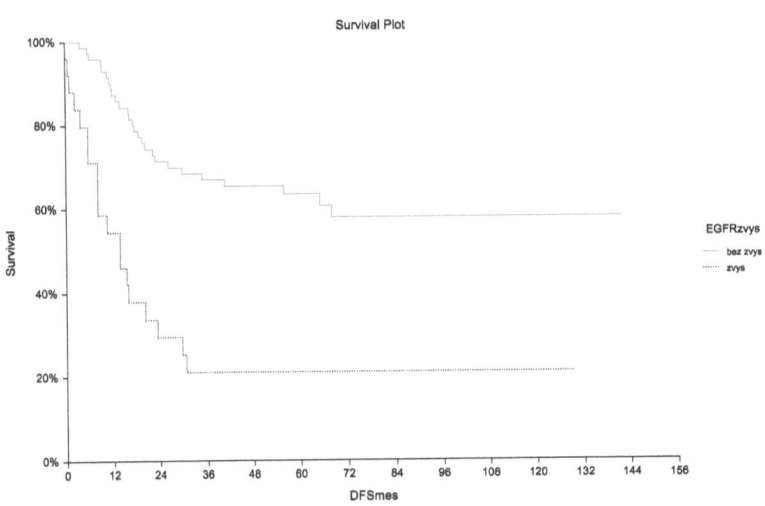

The overexpression of EGFR is observed in 50 – 60 % of rectal carcinoma and is associated with worse prognosis [33 - 35]. Some studies demonstrated the prognostic influence of EGFR expression on outcomes [36 - 43]. On the other hand was published retrospective study that had not demonstrated prognostic influence of EGFR overexpression and K-RAS mutation on OS and DFS in 146 patients with rectal cancer treated by neoadjuvant chemoradiotherapy. In this study was EGFR expression evaluated by in situ hybridization [44]. The most frequently approach of EGFR determination is immunohistochemical (IHC) reaction. This approach was used in most studies. The advantages of IHC determination are simplicity, speed of execution, conservation of tissues morphology. The disadvantages are subjective interpretation by pathologist, existing of more scoring systems to determinate of EGFR expression. The evaluation of EGFR expression is based on percent range, colour intensity, or its combination [39, 41, 55]. Neoadjuvant treatment of rectal cancer has been the topic of several clinical studies I/II phases evaluating the benefits of monoclonal antibodies against EGFR combined with chemotherapy. The chemotherapy regimens included of 5-FU, capecitabine, oxaliplatine or irinotecan. The dose of radiation was in range 45 – 50.4 Gy. The primary point was number of patological completed response as the predictor of longer DFS and OS [65 – 68]. Most dates are for cetuximab than panitumumab. Eleven clinical studies showed average number of pCR only 10.7 % (range 0 – 25 %) of cases [69 – 79]. The explanation of this will need further understanding of the interaction between radiotherapy, EGFR inhibitors, and cytostatics. Initial studies of this topic showed that prolonged exposure of head and neck cancer cells to EGF could increase the effects of radiation [90, 91]. The reason of radiosensitivity was probably through EGF-induces EGFR degradation. Another early studies demonstrated that anti-EGFR antibodies increased radiation-induced apoptosis [92]. Others studies showed the inverse correlation between EGFR expression and response to radiotherapy [93 - 95]. This relationship between EGFR expression and lower response to radiotherapy was confirmed in human head and neck cancer [96]. EGF is known to induce cyclin D1 expression, a protein that is required for progression from the G1 to S phase. Studies of EGFR signalling inhibition have demonstrated proliferation inhibition of cells in G1 phase [25]. EGFR inhibitors commonly produce cytostatic effects rather than cytotoxicity [97, 98]. The interest of new approach combined the EGFR inhibitors and radiation was generated by the experimental studies that demonstrated of radiation-induces EGFR activation in vitro. Confluent cell in culture treated with ionizing radiation rapidly show increased levels of phosphorylated EGFR [99 - 102]. The results is cellular proliferation, DNA-damage repair capability. Phenomenon known as accelerated repopulation. Cetuximab inhibits this radiation-activated of DNAPK, as well as EGFR nuclear import, DNA repair and radiation survival [103]. Various preclinical studies demonstrated that EGFR inhibitors increased radiosensitivity in both in vitr and in vivo [21 – 25, 104, 105]. The important validation of this combination has been from the results of clinical trials in patients with unresectable head and neck cancer. A phase III clinical study, in cohort of 424 patients with locally advanced squamous cell carcinoma of the head and neck, demonstrated the addition of cetuximab to radiotherapy prolonged the median of survival from 28 to 54 months compared with radiotherapy alone. This study represents the first significant success achieved by the addition of an EGFR inhibitors to radiotherapy [82]. The most important role is the interaction between chemotherapy and EGFR inhibitors. Nyati discussed in his review whether the results of the combination of neoadjuvant chemoradiotherapy with EGFR inhibotors could be seen in the suboptimal sequence of administered treatment that might lead to an antagonistic rather than a potentiating effect [106]. Administration of EGFR inhibitors before the cytostatic scan arrested the cell cycle in the G1 phase, which can affect the attenuation of the effects of subsequently administered cytostatics, with an impact on other phases of the cell cycle. It is cytostatics used in the treatment of colorectal cancer (5-FU, capecitabine), that have the most highlighted effect on the cell cycle in the S/G2/M phases of the cell cycle [71]. This would lead to the hypothesis that giving chemotherapy before an EGFR inhibitor would be more effective than reverse schedule. It was published the study that evaluated the optimum sequencing for the combination of gemcitabine and gefitinib. This study demonstrated that gemcitabine followed by gefitinib was superior to the opposite drug order [107]. Another studies showed a similarly results with better effect of sequention cytostatics – EGFR inhibitors than vice versa [108, 109]. It is not clear why the sequence of cytostatics before EGFR inhibitor is crucial in the case of cytotoxic agents that are not necessarily S-phase specific. Another mechanism of interaction cytostatics and EGFR inhibitors is modulation of the EGFR induced pathway. EGFR phosphorylation occurs in response to various cytotoxic drugs, including oxaliplatine, 5-FU, irinotecan [40, 110]. The phosphorylation of EGFR by oxaliplatine or 5-FU treatment alone correlates with the inhibition of cell viability and cell growth by gefitinib [110]. EGFR phosphorylation can lead to the EGFR degardiation and cell dead, under condition of prolonged cellular stress. The reason is s persistent deoxyribonecleaotide pool depletion. The EGFR degradation is dependent of the activation of the proteosome [111]. The other mechanism of synergy between chemotherapy and EGFR inhibitors is through the inhibition of DNA repair. Cytostatics induce various types of DNA damage (strand breaks, DNA adducts, inter- and intra-strand crosslink). The repair of cisplatine induced DNA inter-strand crosslink inhibited by gefitinib [112, 113].

The results of the combination of neoadjuvant treatment and EGFR inhibitors are not successfully [69 - 79]. Similarly EGFR inhibitors not demonstrated better outcomes in adjuvant treatment of colorectal cancer. The phase III clinical study evaluated a total of 2686 patients with colorectal cancer treated with the combination of FOLFOX and cetuximab or FOLFOX alone. The primary aim was overall survival. The addition of cetuximab not demonstrated longer survival compare to chemotherapy alone in median follow-up 28 months

[114]. The other studies evaluating the importance of neoadjuvant or adjuvant treatment with EGFR inhibitors in rectal adenocarcinoma would be performed in future. The study of change of EGFR expression during neoadjuvant chemoradiotherapy is possibility how to better individualised the treatment. Our study would be to define the population of patients with increases of EGFR expression after neoadjuvant chemoradiotherapy. In this group of patients (a total about 25 % of studied patients) it can be assumed that phenomenon acceleration repopulation is applied. This phenomenon is expressed in the smaller number of cases than in patients with squamous cell head and neck cancer. The patients with the increased EGFR expression which would be the benefit form additional therapy anti-EGFR therapy after surgery. Future prospective study could use not only immunohistochemistry ex vivo as in our study, but whole body immunochemistry in vivo by using PET/EGFR. PET detection of EGFR would facilitate the evaluation of EGFR expression not only after, but also during the course of neoadjuvant chemoradiotherapy [115].

In our study we described local relapse in 8 patients that representing 16 %. The CAO/ARO/AIO-94 study comparing neoadjuvant and adjuvant chemoradiotherapy described local relapse in 7.1 % patients [4]. The reason is that in the part of patients not used total mesorectal excision. The significant of TME was conclusively demonstrated in clinical studies [116, 117]. At now presents the TME surgical standard treatment of rectal carcinoma. We further described distant metastases in 17 patients that representing 34 %. The cause is existing of the early subclinical systemic dissemination in the time of diagnosis [118]. This hypothesis confirm the results of clinical studies with approximately 30% incidence of distance metastases [6, 119 - 121].

In our study patients relatively well tolerated the treatment. We not demonstrated the death during the neoadjuvant chemoradotherapy. In 4 patients we stopped of capecitabine administrated for the haematological toxicity. The most common type of toxicity was a gastrointestinal toxicity. This fact is caused by radiation to the pelvic area and adverse events of capecitabine. On other hand the symptoms could be caused by the tumor presence. The rectal carcinoma presents with hemorrhage, tenesmus, pelvic pain, diarrhea. Just this symptoms dominated in patients treated with chemoradiotherapy.

Conclusion

The increase of EGFR expression during neoadjuvant chemoradiotherapy for locally advanced rectal cancer is associated with significant shorter overall survival and disease-free survival.

References

1. Kocáková I, Soumarová R. Chemoradioterapie karcinomu konečníku s 62-72. In: Šlampa P, Soumarová R, Kocáková I et al. Konkomitantní chemoradioterapie solidních nádorů. Nakladatelství Galén 2005, 167 s. ISBN: 80-7262-276-5

2. Gray R, Hills R, Stowe R et al. Adjuvant radiotherapy for rectal cancer: a systemic overview of 8507 patients from 22 randomised trials. Lancet 2001; 358:1291-1304

3. Sauer R, Becker H, Hohenberger W et al. Preoperative versus postoperative chemoradiotherapy for rectal cancer. N Engl J Med 2004; 351: 1731-1740

4. Sauer R, Liersch T, Merkel S et al. Preoperative versus postoperative chemoradiotherapy for rectal cancer: Results of the German CAO/ARO/AIO-94 Randomized Phase III Trial After a Median Follow-up of 11 Years. J Clin Oncol 2012; 30:1926-1933

5. Bosset JF, Collette L, Calais G et al. Chemotherapy with preoperative radiotherapy in rectal cancer. EORTC Radiotherapy Group Trial 22921. N Eng J Med 2006; 355: 1114-1123 Erratum in: N Engl J Med 2007; 357: 728

6. Gerard JP, Conroy T, Bonnetain F et al. Preoperative radiotherapy with or without concurrent fluorouracil and leucovorine in T3-4 rectal cancers: results of FFCD 9203. J Clin Oncol 2006; 24: 4620-4625

7. Ceelen WP, Van Nieuwenhove Y, Fierens K et al. Preoperative chemoradiathion versus radiation alone for stage II and III resectable rectal cancer. Cochrane Database Syst Rev 2009: CD006041

8. Dvořák J, Veselý P, Tomšová M et al. Retrospektivní studie k vyhodnocení výsledků léčby a určení prognostických faktorů u nemocných ozařovaných pro adenokarcinom rekta. Klin Onkol 2006; 19: 187-194

9. Dvořák J, Richter I, Buka D et al. Chemoradioterapie lokálně pokročilých karcinomů rekta. Kolorektální karcinom 2013, Farmakoterapie suppl. 2013; 42-46

10. Sirák I, Hatlová J, Petera J et al. Receptor pro epidermální růstový faktor a jeho úloha v radioterapii. Klin Okol 2008; 21: 338-347

11. Willett CG, Duda DG, Czito BG et al. Targeted therapy in rectal cancer. Oncology 2007; 21: 1055-1065

12. Yarden Y. The EGFR family and its ligands in human cancer: signalling mechanism and therapeutic opportunities. Eur J Cancer 2001; 37: S3-S8

13. Uberall I, Kolar Z, Trojec R et al. The status and role of ErbB receptors in human cancer. Exp Mol Pathol 2008; 84: 79-89

14. Yarden Y, Sliwkowski MX. Untangling the ErbB signalling network. Nat Rev Mol Cell Biol 2001; 2: 127-137

15. Lin SY, Makino K, Xia W et al. Nuclear localization of EGF receptor and its potential new role as a transcription factor. Nat Cell Biol 2001; 3: 802-808

16. Oksvold MP, Huitfeldt H, Stang E et al. Localizing the EGF receptor. Nat Cell Biol 2002; 4: E22-23

17. Waugh MG, Hsuan JJ. EGF receptors as transcription factors: ridiculous or sublime? Nat Cell Biol 2001; 3: E209-E211

18. Walther A, Johnstone E, Swanton C et al. Genetics prognostic and predictive markers in colorectal cancer. Nat Rev Canc 2009; 9: 489-499

19. Akimoto T, Hunter NR, Buchmiller L et al. Inverse relationship between epidermal growth factor expression and radiocurability of murine carcinomas. Clin Cancer Res 1999; 5: 2884-2890

20. Liang K, Ang KK, Milas L et al. The epidermal growth factor receptor mediates radioresistance. Int J Radiat Biol Phys 2003; 57: 246-254

21. Verbeek BS, Andriaansen-Slot SS, Vroom TM et al. Overexpression of EGFR and c-erbB2 causes enhanced cell migration in human breast cancer cells and NIH3T3 fibroblasts. FEBS Lett 1998; 425: 145-150

22. Withers HR. The 4 R's of radiotherapy. In: J. T. Lett and H. Alder (eds.), Advances in Radiation Biology, Vol. 5, str. 241-271. New York: Academic Press, 1975

23. Bandyopathy D, Mandal M, Adam L et al. Physical interaction between epidermal growth factor receptor and DNA-dependent protein kinase in mammalian cells. J Biol Chem 1998; 273: 1568-1573

24. Meyn RE, Munshi A, Haymach JV et al. Receptor signalling as a regulatory mechanism of DNA repair. Radiother Oncol 2009; 92: 316-322

25. Chinnaiyan P, Huang S, Vallabhaneni G et al. Mechanism of enhanced radiation response following epidermal growth factor receptor signaling inhibition by erlotinib (Tarceva). Cancer Res 2005; 65: 3328-35

26. Lammering G, Valerie K, Lin PS et al. Radiosensitization of malignant glioma cells through overexpression of dominant negative epidermal growth factor receptor. Clin Cancer Reserch 2001; 6: 2166-2174

27. Withers HR, Taylor JM, Maciejewski B et al. The hazard of accelerated tumour clonogen repopulation during radiotherapy. Acta Oncol 1988; 27: 131-146

28. Baumann M, Petersen C, Eichler W et al. Mechanism of repopulation in experimental squamos cell carcinoma. In: Kogelnik HD, Lukas P, Sedlmayer F. Progress in radiation-oncology, vol.7. Bologna, Monduzzi; 2002, s. 417-422

29. Begg AC. Prediction of repopulation rates and radiosensitivity in human tumours. Int J Radiat Biol 1994; 65: 103-108

30. Fowler JF. Rapid repopulation in radiotherapy: a debate on mechanism. The phantom of tumor treatment-continually rapid proliferation inmasked. Radiother Oncol 1991; 22: 156-158

31. Schmitdt-Ullrich RK, Contessa JN, Dent P et al. Molecular mechanism of radiation-induced accelerated repopulation. Radiat Oncol Investig 1999; 7: 321-330

32. Huang SM, Harari PM. Modulation of radiation response after epidermal growth factor receptor blockade in squamous cell carcinomas: inhibition of damage repair, cell cycle kinetics, and tumor angiogenesis. Clin Cancer Res 2000; 6: 2166-2174

33. Steele RJ, Kelly P, Ellul B et al. Epidermal growth factor receptor expression in colorectal cancer. Br J Surg 1990; 77: 1352-1354

34. Mayer A, Takimoto M, Fritz E et al. The prognostic significance of proliferating cell nuclear antigen, epidermal growth factor receptor, and MDR gene expression in colorectal cancer. Cancer 1993; 71: 2454-2460

35. Khorana AA, Ryan CK, Cox C et al. Vascular enndothelial growth factor, CD68, and epidermal growth factor receptor expression and survival in patients with stage II and stage III colon carcinoma: a role for the host response in prognosis. Cancer 2003; 97: 960-968

36. Azria D, Bibeau F, Barbier N et al. Prognostic impact of epidermal growth factor receptor (EGFR) expression on loco-regional recurrence after preoperative radiotherapy in rectal cancer. BMC Cancer 2005; 5: 62

37. Shengjin L, Jae-Sung K, Jin-man K et al. Epidermal growth factor receptor as a prognostic factor in locally advanced rectal-cancer patiens treated with preoperative chemoradiation. Int J Radiat Oncol Biol Phys 2006; 65: 705-712

38. Giralt J, de las Heras M, Cerezo L et al. The expression of epidermal growth factor receptor results in a worse prognosis for patients with rectal cancer treated with preoperative radiotherapy. Radiother Oncol 2005; 74: 101-108

39. Kopp R, Rothbauer E, Ruge M et al. Clinical implications of the EGF receptor ligand system for tumour progression and survival in gastrointestinal carcinomas: evidence for new therapeutic options. Recent Results Cancer Res 2003; 162: 115-132

40. Li S, Kim JS, Kim JM et al. Epidermal growth factor receptor as a prognostic factor in locally advanced rectal cancer patiens treated with preoperative chemoradiation. Int J Radiat Oncol Biol Phys 2006; 65: 1019-1028

41. Kim JS, Kim JM, Li S al. Epidermal growth factor receptor as a predictor of tumour downstaging in locally advanced rectal cancer patients treated with preoperative radiotherapy. Int J Radiat Cncol Biol Phys 2006; 66: 195-200

42. Bertolini F, Bengala C, Losi L et al. Prognostic and predictive value of baseline and post-treatment molecular marker expression in locally advanced rectal cancer treated with neoadjuvant chemoradiotherapy. Int J Radiat Oncol Biol Phys 2007; 68: 1455-68

43. Zlobec I, Vuong T, Compton CC et al. Combined analysis of VEGF and EGFR predicts complete tumour response in rectal cancer treated with preoperative radiotherapy. Br J Cancer 2008; 98: 450-456

44. Bengala C, Bettelli S, Bertolini F et al. Prognostic role of EGFR gene copy number and KRAS mutation in patients with locally advanced rectal cancer treated with preoperative chemoradiotherapy. Brit J of Canc 2010; 103: 1019-1024

45. Marquardt F, Rödel F, Capalbo G et al. Molecular targeted treatment and radiation therapy for rectal cancer. Strahlenther Onkol 2009; 185: 371-378

46. Baumann M, Grégoire V. Molecular-targeted agents for enhancing tumour response, s. 287-300. In: Joiner M, van der Kogel A: Basic Clinical Radiobiology. 4th ed. London, Edward Arnold, 2009, 375 s

47. Shepherd FA., Pereira JR., Ciuleanu T et al. Erlotinib in Previously treated Non-Small-Cell Lung Cancer. N Engl J Med 2005, 353: 123-132

48. Johnson S, Piplej J, Pivot X et al. Lapatinib combined with letrozole versus letrozole and placebo as first-line therapy for postmenopausal hormone receptor-positive metastatic breast cancer. J Clin Oncol 2009; 28:1-11

49. Rothenberg ML, LaFleur B, Levy DE et al. Randomized phase II trial of the clinical and biological effects of two dose levels of gefitinib in patients with recurrent colorectal adenocarcinoma. J Clin Oncol 2005; 23: 9265 – 9274

50. Meyerhardt JA, Zhu AX, Enzinger PC et al. Phase II study of capecitabine, oxaliplatine, and erlotinib in previously treated patiens with metastatic colorectal cancer. J Clin Oncol 2006; 24: 1892-1897

51. Townsley CA, Major P, Siu LL et al. Phase II study of erlotinib (OSI-774) in patiens with metastatic colorectal cancer. Br J Cancer 2006; 94: 1136-1143

52. Van Cutsem E, Verslype C, Beale P et al. A phase Ib dose-escalation study of erlotinib, capecitabine and oxaliplatine in metastatic colorectal cancer patiens. Ann Oncol 2008; 19: 332-339

53. Williams KJ, Telfer BA, Stratford IJ et al. ZD1839 (Iressa), a specific oral epidermal growth factor receptor tyrosine kinase inhibitor potentiates radiohterapy in a human colorectal cancer xenograft model. Br J Cancer 2002; 86: 1157-1161

54. Valentini V, De Paoli A, Gambacorta MA et al. Infusional 5-fluorouracil and ZD 1839 (gefitinib – Iressa) in combination with preoperative radiotherapy in patiens with locally advanced rectal cancer: a phase I and II trial (1839IL/0092). Int J Radiat Oncol Biol Phys 2008; 72: 644-649

55. Cunningham D, Humblet Y, Siena S et al. Cetuximab monotherapy and cetuximab plus irinotekan in irinotekan-refractory metastatic colorectal cancer. N Engl J Med 2004; 351: 337-345

56. Finocchiaro G, Capuzzo F, Janne PA et al. EGFR HER2, and K-ras as predictive factors for cetuximab sensitivity in colorectal cancer. Proc Am Soc Clin Oncol 2007; 25: 168s Abstract 4021

57. Van Cutsem E, Kohne CH, Láng I et al. Cetuximab plus irinotecan, fluorouracil, and leucovorine as fist-line treatment for metastatic colorectal cancer: update analysis of overall survival according to tumor KRAS and BRAF station status. J Clin Oncol 2011; 29: 2011-2019

58. Bokemeyer C, Bondarenko I, Makhson A et al. Fluorouracil, leucovorin, and oxaliplatin with and without cetuximab in the first-line treatment of metastatic colorectal cancer. J Clin Oncol 2009; 27: 663-671

59. Maugham TS, Adams RA, Smith CG et al. Addition of cetuximab to oxaliplatine-based first-line combination chemotherapy for treatment of advanced colorectal cancer: results of the randomised phase 3 MRC COIN trial. Lancet 2011; 377: 2013-2114

60. Tveit KM, Guren T, Glimelius B et al. Phase III trial of cetuximab with continuous or intermittent fluorouracil, luecovorine, and oxaliplatine (Nordic FLOX) versus FLOX alone in

first-line treatment of metstatic colorectal cancer: the NORDIC-VII study. J Clin Oncol 2012; 30: 1755-1762

61. Van Cutsem E, Peeters M, Siena S et al. Open.label phase III trial of panitumumab plus bets supportive care compared with best supportive care alone in patiens with chemotherapy-refractory metastatic colorectal cancer. J Clin Oncol 2007; 25: 1658-1664

62. Oliner KS, Douillard JY, Siena S et al. Analysis of KRAS/NRAS and BRAF station in the phase III PRIME study of panitumumab (pmab) plus FOLFOX versus FOLFOX as first-line treatment (tx) for metastatic colorectal cancer (mCRC). J Clin Oncol 2013; 31(Suppl): Abstract 3511

63. Ince WL, Jubb AM, Holden SN et al. Association of k-ras, b-raf, and p53 status with the treatment effect of bevacizumab. J Natl Cancer Inst 2005; 97: 981-989

64. Richman SD, Seymour MT, Cahmbers P et al. KRAS and BRAF mutations in advanced colorectal cancer are associated with poor prognosis but not preclude bendit form oxaliplatin or irinotecan: results from the MRC FOCUS trial. J Clin Oncol 2009; 27: 5931-5937

65. Rödel C, Martus P, Papadoupolos T et al. Prognostic significance of tumor regression after preoperative chemoradiotherapy for rectal cancer. J Clin Oncol. 2005; 23: 8688-8696

66. Janjan NA, Crane C, Feig BW et al. Improved overall survival among responders to preoperative chemoradiation for locally advanced rectal cancer. Am J Clin Oncol. 2001; 24: 107-112

67. Janjan NA, Abbruzzese J, Pazdur R et al. Prognostic implications of response to preoperative infusional chemoradiation in locally advanced rectal cancer. Radiother Oncol. 1999; 51: 153-160

68. Maas M, Nelemans PJ, Valentini V et al. Long-term outcome in patients with a pathological complete response after chemoradiation for rectal cancer: a pooled analysis of indivudual patient data. Lancet Oncol. 2010; 11: 835-844

69. Chung KY, Minsky B, Schrag D et al. Phase I trial of preoperative cetuximab with concurrent continuous infusion 5-fluorouracil and pelvic radiation in patients with local-regionally advanced rectal cancer. J Clin Oncol 2006; 24 (18 suppl): Abstract 3560

70. Machiels JP, Sempoux C, Scalliet P et al. Phase I/II study of preoperative cetuximab, capecitabine, and external beam radiotherapy in patients with rectal cancer. Ann Oncol 2007; 18: 738-744

71. Rödel C, Arnold D, Hipp M et al. Phase I-II trial of cetuximab, capecitabine, oxaliplatin, and radiotherapy as preoperative treatment in rectal cancer. Int J Radiat Oncol Biol Phys 2008; 70: 1081-1086

72. Hofheinz RD, Horisberger K, Woernle C et al. Phase I trial of cetuximab in combination with capecitabine, weekly irinotecan, and radiotherapy as neoadjuvant therapy for rectal cancer. Int J Radiat Oncol Biol Phys 2006; 66: 1384 – 1390

73. Horisberger K, Treschl A, Mai S et al. Cetuximab in combination with capecitabine, irinotecan, and radiotherapy for patients with locally advanced rectal cancer: results of a Phase II MARGIT trial. Int J Radiat Oncol Biol Phys 2009; 74: 1487-1493

74. Bertolini F, Chiara S, Bengala C et al. Neoadjuvant treatment with single-agent cetuximab followed by 5-FU, cetuximab, and pelvic radiotherapy: a phase II study in locally advanced rectal cancer. Int J Radiat Oncol Biol Phys 2009; 73: 466-472

75. Hong YS, Kim DY, Lee KS et al. Phase II study of preoperative chemoradiation (CRT) witj cetuximab, irinotecan and capecitabine in patiens with locally advanced resectable rectal cancer. J Clin Oncol 2007; 25: 18S:174s (abstrakt 4045)

76. Cabebe EC, Kuo T, Koong M et al. Phase I trial of preoperative cetuximab in combination with oxaliplatine, capecitabine, and radiation therapy for locally advanced rectal cancer. J Clin Oncol 2008; 26 (suppl) abstrakt 15019

77. Eisterer WM, De Vries A, Oefner D et al. Neoadjuvant chemoradiation therapy with capecitabine plus cetuximab and external beam radiotherapy in locally advanced rectal cancer (LARC) ABCSG trial R03. J Clin Oncol 2009; 27:15S(part I of II) 195s (abstract 4109)

78. Velenik V, Ocvirk J, Oblak I et al. Neoadjuvant cetuximab, capecitabine, and radiotherapy (RT) in locally advanced resectable rectal cancer: results of a phase II trial. J Clin Oncol 2009; 27: (abstrakt e15029)

79. Kim SY, Hong YS, Kim DY et al. Preoperative chemoradiation with cetuximab, irinotecan, and capecitabine in patients with locally advanced resectable rectal cancer: a multicenter phase II study. Int J Radiat Oncol Biol Phys 2011; 81: 677-683

80. Hartley A, Ho KF, McConkey C et al. Pathological complete response following preoperative chemoradiotherapy in rectal cancer: analysis of phase II/III trials. Br J Radiol 2005; 78: 934-938

81. Pinto C, Di Fabio F, Maiello E et al. Phase II study of panitumumab, oxaliplatin, 5-fluorouracil, and concurrent radiotherapy as preoperative treatment in high-risk locally advanced rectal cancer patients (StarPan/STAR-02 Study). Ann Oncol 2011; 22: 2424-2430

82. Bonner JA, Harari PM, Giralt J et al. Radiotherapy plus cetuximab for squamos-cell carcinoma of head and neck. N Engl J Med 2006; 354:567-578

83. Dewdney A, Cunningham D, Tabernero J et al. Multicenter randomized phase II clinical trial comparing neoadjuvant oxaliplatin, capecitabine, and preoperative radiotherapy with or without cetuximab followed by total mesorectal excision in patients with high-risk rectal cancer (EXPERT-C). J Clin Oncol 2012; 30:1620-1627

84. Bengala C, Bettelli S, Bertolini F et al. Epidermal growth factor receptor gene copy number, K-ras station and pathological response to preoperative cetuximab, 5-FU and radiation therapy in locally advanced rectal cancer. Ann Oncol 2009; 20: 469-474

85. Debucquoy A, Haustermans K, Daemen A et al. Molecular response to cetuximab and efficacy of preoperative cetuximab-based chemoradiation in rectal cancer. J Clin Oncol 2009; 27: 2751-2757

86. Luna-Pérez P, Segura J, Alvarado I et al. Specific c-K-ras gene station as a tumour-response marker in locally advanced rectal cancer trated with preoperative chemoradiotherapy. Ann Surg Oncol 2000; 7: 727-731

87. Hirvikoski P, Auvinen A, Cummings B et al. K-ras and p53 mutations and overexpressions as prognostic factors in fiale rectal carcinoma. Anticancer Res 1999;19: 685-691

88. Dvořák J, Sitorová V, Ryška A et al. The prognostic significance of changes of tumour epidermal growth factor receptor expression after neoadjuvant chemoradiation in patiens with rectal adenocarcinoma. Strahlenter Onkol 2012; 10: 145-147

89. Richter I, Dvořák J, Blüml A, Čermáková E, Bartoš J, Urbanec M, Sitorová V, Ryška A, Sirák I, Buka D, Ferko A, Melichar B, Petera J. Vliv předoperační chemoradioterapie na změnu exprese epidermálního růstového faktoru u pacientů léčených předoperační chemoradioterapií pro lokálně pokročilý karcinom rekta. Klin Onkol 2014; 27:361-366

90. Kwok TT, Sutherland RM. Enhacement of sensitivity of human squamous carcinoma cells to radiation by epidermal growth factor receptor. J Natl Cancer Inst 1989; 81:1020-1024

91. Bonner JA, Maihle NJ, Folven BR et al. The interaction of epidermal growth factor and radiation in human head and neck squamous cell carcinoma cell lines with vastly different radiosensitivities. Int J Radiat Oncol Biol Phys 1994; 29:243-247

92. Balaban N, Moni J, Shannon M et al. The eefect of ionizing radiation on signal transduction: Antibodies to EGF receptor sensitize A431 cells to radiation. Biochim Biophys Acta 1996; 1314:147-156

93. Sheridan MT, O'Dwyer T, Seymour CB et al. Potencial indicators of radiosenzitivity in squamous cell carcinoma of hte head and neck. Radiat Oncol Invstig 1997; 5:180-186

94. Akimoto T, Hunter NR, Buchmiller L et al. Inverse relationship between epidermal growth factor receptor expression and radiocurability of murine carcinomas. Clin Cancer Res 1999; 5:2884-2890

95. Milas L, Fan Z, Andratschke NH et al. Epidermal growth factor receptor and tumour response to radiation: in vivo preclinical studies. Int J Rad Oncol Biol Phys 2004; 58:966-971

96. Ang KK, Berkey BA, Tu X et al. Impact of epidermal growth factor receptor expression on survival and pattern of relapse in patiens with advanced head and neck carcinoma. Cancer Res 2002; 62:7350-7356

97. Peng D, Fan Z, Lu Y et al. Anti-epidermal growth factor receptor monoclonal antibody 225 upregulates p27KIP1 and induces G1 arrest in prostatic cancer cell line DU 145. Cancer Res 1996; 56:3666-3669

98. Di Gennaro E, Barbarino M, Bruzzese F et a. Critical role of both p27KIP1 and p21CIP1/WAF1 in the antiproliferative effect of ZH 1839 (Iressa), an epidermal growth factor

receptor tyrosin kinase inhibitor, in head and neck squamous carcinoma cells. J Cell Physiol 2003; 195:139-150

99.Schmitd-Ullrich RK, Valerie K, Foglman PB et al. Radiation-induced autophosphorylation of epidermal growth factor receptor in human malignat mammay and squamous epithelial cells. Radiat Res 1996; 145:81-85

100. Schmitd-Ullrich RK, Mikkelsen RB, Dent P et al. Radiation-induced prolifaration of the human A431 squamous carcinoma cell is dependent on EGFR tyrosine phosphorylation. Oncogene 1997; 15:1191-1197

101.Dent P, Reardon DB, Park JS et al. Radiation-induced release of transforming growth factor receptor and mitogen-activated protein kinase pathway in carcinoma cells, leading to increased proliferation and protection from radiation-induced cell dead. Mol Biol Cell 1999; 10: 2493-2506

102.Contessa JN, Hampton J, Lammerking G et al. Ionizing radiation activates Erb-B receptor dependent Akt and p70 S6 kinase signalling in carcinoma cells. Oncogene 2002; 21:4032-4041

103.Dittmann K. Mayer C, Fehrenbacher B et al. Radiation-induced epidermal growth factor receptor nuclear import is linked to activation of DNA-dependent protein kinase. J Biol Chem 2005; 280:31182-31189

104. Milas L, Mason K, Hunter N et al. In vivo enhancement of tumour radioresponse by C225 antiepidermal growth factor receptor antibody. Clin Cancer Res 200; 6:701-708

105. Nyati MK, Maheshwari D, Hanasoqe S et al. Radiosensitization by pan ErbB inhibitor CI-1033 in vitro and in vivo. Clin Cancer Res 2004; 10:691-700

106. Nyati MK, Morgan MA, Feng FY et al. Integration of EGFR inhibitors with radiochemotherapy. Nat Rev Cancer 2006; 6: 876-885

107.Chun PY, Feng FY, Scheuer AM et al. Synergistic effects of gemcitabine and gefitinib in the treatment of head and neck carcinoma. Cancer Res 2006; 66:981-988

108.Azzariti A, Xu JM, Porcelli L et al. The schedule-dependent enhanced cytotoxic activity of 7-ethyl-10-hydroxy.camptothecin (SN-38) in combination with Gefitinib (Iresa, ZD 1839). Biochem Pharmacol 2004; 68: 135-144

109. Xu J, Azzariti A, Severino M et al. Characterization of sequence-dependent synergy between ZD 1839 (Iressa) and oxaliplatine. Biochem Pharmacol 2003; 66:551-563

110. Van Schaeybroeck S, Karaiskou-McCaul A, Kelly D et al. Epidermal growth factor receptor activity determines response of colorectal cancer cells to gefitinib alone and in combination with chemotherapy. Clin Cancer Res 2005; 11: 7480-7489

111. Feng FY. EGFR degradation: a novel mechanism of gemcitanine-induces cell dech: in head and neck cancer cell lines. In 14th SPORE investagators workshop 154, Baltimore 2006

112. Friedmann B, Caplin M, Hartley JA et al. Modulation of DNA repair in vitra after treatment with chemotherapeutic agents by the epidermal growth factor receptor inhibitor gefitinib (ZD 1839). Clin Cancer Res 2004; 10: 6476-6486

113. Friedmann B, Caplin M, Savic B et al. Interaction of the epidermal growth factor receptor and the DNA-dependent protein kinase pathway following gefitinib treatment. Mol Cancer Ther 2006; 5:209-218

114. Alberts SR, Sargent DJ, Nair S et al. Effect of oxaliplatine, fluorouracil, and leucovorine with or without cetuximab on survival among patiens with resected stage III colon cancer: a randomised trial. JAMA 2012; 307:1383-1393

115. Mishani E, Abourbeh G. Cancer molecular imaging: radionuclide-based biomarkers of the epidermal growth factor receptor (EGFR). Curr Top Med Chem 2007; 7: 1755-1772

116. Folkesson J, Birgisson H, Pahlman L et al. Swedisch Rectal cancer Trial: long lasting benefits from radiotherapy on survival and local recurence rate. J Clin Oncol 2005; 23: 5644-5650

117. Kapiteijn E, Marijnen CA, Nagtegaal ID et al. Preoperative radiotherapy combined with total mesorectal excision for resectable rectal cancer. N Engl J Med 2001; 345: 6386 – 6346

118. De Caluwé L, van Nieuwenhove Y, Ceelen WP et al. Preoperative chemoradiation versus radiation alone for stage II and III resectable rectal cancer. Cochrane Database Syst Rev 2013; 2:CD006041

119. Bosset JF, Collette L, Calais G et al. Chemotherapy with preoperative radiotherapy in rectal cancer. N Engl J Med 2006; 355: 1114-1123

120. Boulis-Wassif S, Gerard A, Loygue J et al. Final results of a randomized trial on the treatment of rectal cancer with preoperative radiotherapy alone or in combination with 5-fluorouracil, followed by radical surgery. Trial of the european Organization on Research and Treatment of Cancer Gastroninestinal Tract Cancer Group. Cancer 1984; 53: 1811-1818

121. Bujko K, Nowacki MP, Nasierowska-Guttmejer A et al. Long-term results of a randomized trial comparing preoperative short-course radiotherapy with preoperative conventionally fractionated chemoradiation for rectal cancer. Br J Surg 2006; 93: 1215-1223

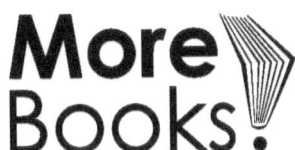
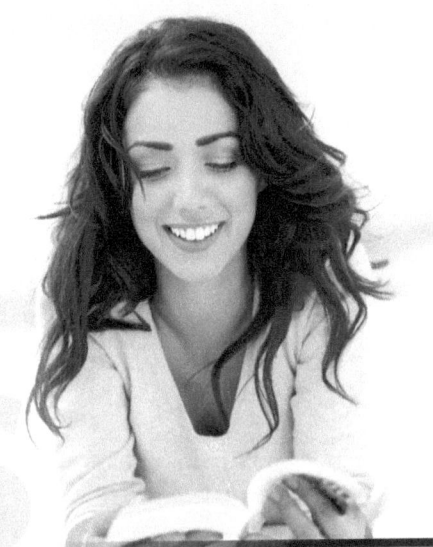

I want morebooks!

Buy your books fast and straightforward online - at one of the world's fastest growing online book stores! Environmentally sound due to Print-on-Demand technologies.

Buy your books online at
www.get-morebooks.com

Kaufen Sie Ihre Bücher schnell und unkompliziert online – auf einer der am schnellsten wachsenden Buchhandelsplattformen weltweit! Dank Print-On-Demand umwelt- und ressourcenschonend produziert.

Bücher schneller online kaufen
www.morebooks.de

OmniScriptum Marketing DEU GmbH
Heinrich-Böcking-Str. 6-8
D - 66121 Saarbrücken
Telefax: +49 681 93 81 567-9

info@omniscriptum.com
www.omniscriptum.com

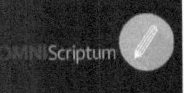